# UNDERSTANDING

# GINSENG

# AND BENEFITS

## A Comprehensive Guide to Understanding Its Major Targets, Focus, Optimal Well-being and Key Points

## DR. LACEY MICHELLE

Copyright © Lacey Michelle 2023

all rights reserved. No part of this book may be reproduced, stored in a retrieval system, or transmitted in any form or by any means electronic, mechanical, photocopy, recording, or any other without prior written permission from the author, except for brief quotations in critical reviews or articles.

# Disclaimer:

The information provided in this book is for general informational purposes only and is not intended as medical advice.

Readers are encouraged to consult with a qualified healthcare professional for any health concerns or questions.

The author of this book is not affiliated with any individual, website, organization, or products mentioned within.

This book does not endorse or promote any specific brands, services, or external entities. Any references made are purely for illustrative purposes and should not be construed as endorsements.

Readers are responsible for their own decisions and should conduct their own research before making any health-related choices.

Any liability resulting from the use of this information, whether direct or indirect, is disclaimed by the author and publisher.

# Contents

First Off

As a supplement, ginseng offers an engrossing dive into the world of this age-old herb and its cultural and historical significance. This thorough book delves deeply into the subject of ginseng, highlighting its historical significance and identifying the several varieties that have fascinated people for ages.

The Ginseng Types

We begin by being introduced to the three main types of ginseng: Siberian, American, and Asian ginseng. For individuals looking to reap the benefits, each variety offers a diverse range of possibilities due to its distinct qualities and attributes.

The Nutritional Profile of Ginseng

The nutritional profile of ginseng is a major area of study, revealing the amazing variety of chemicals and nutrients it contains. This section also reveals the numerous health advantages of ginseng use, highlighting how it may improve wellbeing.

## Ginseng as a Conventional Therapy

Next, we delve into the domain of customs, examining the centuries-old use of ginseng in diverse cultures. This mysterious herb is the subject of folklore and legends; this part explores the fascinating tales and customs that have developed around it.

## Effects of Ginseng on Health

The health benefits of ginseng are many and include immune system support, higher energy, improved cognitive function, and less stress. We explore ginseng's adaptogenic qualities and highlight how it can be used as a general health enhancer.

Ginseng in Contemporary Medicine:

Scientific studies have shown ginseng's potential medicinal uses. We discuss the most recent research, possible uses in contemporary medicine, and safe and efficient dose recommendations in this area.

Selecting the Best Supplement for Ginseng

Choosing the best ginseng supplement might be difficult. We discuss several types of ginseng supplements and offer advice on factors related to purity and quality.

Including Ginseng in Your Daily Routine

The benefits of ginseng go beyond pills. Discover how to include ginseng into your everyday routine with mouthwatering dishes, age-old healing methods, and advice on holistic health.

Ginseng for Skincare and Beauty

Learn the benefits of ginseng for glowing skin and glossy hair. Discover the world of DIY ginseng cosmetics and how this plant can improve your regimen for skincare.

Ginseng for Everyday Health

This section looks at how ginseng can be consumed regularly in the form of dietary supplements and drinks like ginseng tea. Discover all the ways this amazing herb can improve your daily well-being.

Agriculture of Ginseng and Sustainability

We explore the nuances of ginseng cultivation and sustainable methods to guarantee its long-term availability for those who are interested in doing so.

Ginseng and Overall Health

We emphasize how ginseng works well with other supplements and how it can help lead a peaceful and healthy lifestyle.

In summary

As our exploration of ginseng as a supplement comes to an end, we look forward to what this amazing herb has in store. We hope that our concluding remarks and suggestions will act as a compass for anyone considering ginseng as a way to enhance their health and vigor.

# CHAPTER ONE

## The Universe Of Ginseng

### History And Origin:

With origins in Eastern Asia, ginseng is a popular herbal supplement with a long history dating back centuries, and it is well known for its possible health advantages. Because of its human-like form, the Chinese term "ren shen," which translates to "man root" or "essence of man," is where the word "ginseng" originates. The use of ginseng dates back thousands of years to Native American, Chinese, and Korean cultures.

The belief in the revitalizing and healing benefits of ginseng is the reason for its use in history. Ginseng is regarded by traditional Chinese medicine (TCM) as a potent adaptogen, or a herb that aids the body in adjusting to a variety of stimuli, both mental and physical. About 2000 years ago, Shen Nong Ben Cao Jing, one of the earliest Chinese pharmaceutical writers, made the first known mention of it.

Ginseng comes in a variety of forms, each with distinct qualities and origins in different parts of the world. The most well-known types are as follows:

Asian ginseng (Panax ginseng): Native to China, Siberia, and Korea, this variety of ginseng is also known as Korean ginseng. Its energizing and invigorating qualities have long been recognized. Asian ginseng is further divided into red and white varieties, the latter of which is dried and steamed.

Native Americans prized American ginseng (Panax quinquefolius), which subsequently became well-known in traditional Chinese medicine. American ginseng is a native of North America. It is typically used to relieve tension and encourage relaxation. It is thought to as a softer, cooler variety of ginseng.

Eleutherococcus senticosus, sometimes known as Siberian ginseng, is not a real ginseng although it does have some similar adaptogenic qualities. Native to Russia and other regions of Asia, it has long been utilized for its immune-stimulating and stamina-boosting properties.

Japanese ginseng, or Panax japonicus, is prized in the local culture for its possible health advantages but is less well-known abroad. It is native to Japan.

Notoginseng (Panax notoginseng): This variety of ginseng is mostly farmed in China's

Yunnan province and is well-known for its possible anti-inflammatory and cardiovascular benefits.

Selecting the type of ginseng that best suits your health objectives is crucial because they all contain unique bioactive components and may have differing health advantages.

Cultural Significance of Ginseng: Throughout history, ginseng has been integral to the customs and cultures of many different societies. A plant with a rich mythological and folkloric history, ginseng is frequently referred to be the "king of herbs" in traditional Chinese medicine. Regular consumption of it was thought to provide longevity, vitality, and knowledge to its users. Ginseng was also thought to represent the Yin and Yang energies working together harmoniously to balance the body's essential forces.

Ginseng is closely associated with Korean culture and has long been seen as a sign of success, good fortune, and wealth. In South Korea, ginseng is a well-liked present, especially for ceremonies and special events.

American ginseng was highly valued and traditionally used for its therapeutic qualities in Native American societies. It was frequently exchanged with early European settlers and used in their herbal treatments.

The cultural relevance of ginseng is not limited to Asia or North America.

 Due to its widespread use as an adaptogen and natural treatment, it is now considered a great herbal supplement.

As a result of its continued significance in the fields of herbal medicine and nutrition, ginseng is now a highly sought-after element in the worldwide health and wellness sector and is still incorporated into many facets of modern culture.

## The Health Benefits Of Ginseng

The perennial herb ginseng, which is native to both Asia and North America, has a long history of usage in herbal and traditional Chinese and Korean medicine.

This amazing plant is well-known for its many health advantages, which have made it a popular supplement in the natural medicine industry. Ginseng is a multipurpose plant that has many positive effects on human health.

# CHAPTER TWO

## The Medicinal Properties Of Ginseng

Often called an adaptogen, ginseng aids in the body's ability to adjust to stress and preserve equilibrium. The component of the ginseng plant that is most frequently utilized in herbal remedies is the root. Ginsenosides are bioactive chemicals found in it, and they are thought to be the source of many of its therapeutic qualities. Due to its anti-inflammatory, antioxidant, and neuroprotective properties, ginseng is frequently used to treat a wide range of health problems, including stress, exhaustion, and sexual dysfunction.

Immune Support and Ginseng

Immune system stimulation is one of ginseng's most well-known advantages. It has been demonstrated that the ginsenosides in ginseng increase immune cell function and strengthen the body's resistance to infections. This characteristic is very helpful in avoiding common colds and flu seasons. Ginseng is thought to lessen the likelihood of illness by enhancing the body's ability to fend against infections.

## The Function Of Ginseng In Vigor And Energy

Ginseng is often used to fight weariness and boost vitality in general. This is explained by its ability to boost endurance and enhance the body's capacity to use energy more effectively.

If you're a professional athlete searching for a natural way to boost your performance or just someone hoping to fight off everyday fatigue, ginseng can be a useful ally in boosting your energy and stamina.

## Improved Cognitive Function With Ginseng

Ginseng's ability to improve cognitive function has drawn attention. It is thought to improve focus, memory, and mental sharpness. According to research, ginsenosides can shield brain tissue from oxidative stress and inflammation, two things that might lead to cognitive deterioration. Because of this, ginseng is frequently regarded as a natural remedy for improving cognitive performance and maybe averting illnesses like Alzheimer's disease.

## Ginseng As A Stress Reduction Tool

Modern life is full of stress, and ginseng has been used for generations to lessen the negative effects of stress. As an adaptogen, ginseng controls the release of stress chemicals like cortisol, which helps the body handle stress. This may result in less anxiety, happier feelings, and an increased ability to handle daily pressures with resilience. To control their stress levels and preserve their sense of well-being, many people take ginseng supplements.

The health advantages of ginseng are numerous and varied. This herbal therapy has many benefits, including immunological support, energy boosting, improved cognition, and stress control. Before adding ginseng supplements to your daily regimen, you should speak with a healthcare provider, though, as individual reactions and possible drug interactions can differ. Natural health and well-being continue to be interested in ginseng because of its rich history and potential medical benefits.

The intriguing and popular herbal supplement ginseng is well-known for its possible health advantages. Ginseng comes in a variety of forms, each having special qualities and possible therapeutic uses. Some of the most well-known ginseng varieties will be covered in this article, along with lesser-known ones like Panax, American, and Siberian ginseng.

Panax Ginseng:

 Also referred to as Asian or Korean ginseng, Panax ginseng is arguably the most well-known and well-researched type of ginseng. For thousands of years, it has been a part of traditional Chinese medicine. The putative adaptogenic qualities of Panax ginseng are well-known; these qualities may aid the body in adjusting to stress and bolster general resilience. It is thought to increase vitality, lessen weariness, and enhance mental clarity. Supplementing with Panax ginseng helps a lot of people maintain their physical and emotional health.

Panax quinquefolius, or American ginseng, is another well-known variation. It is native to North America and has been utilized for generations by Native American cultures. American ginseng has a reputation for having relaxing and stress-relieving properties. According to certain research, it might aid in enhancing mental clarity and lessening the harmful effects of stress on the body. It's frequently used to boost immunity and encourage relaxation.

Eleutherococcus senticosus, sometimes known as Siberian ginseng, is sometimes referred to as real ginseng despite lacking the same adaptogenic qualities. Native to Siberia and other Asian regions is this herb. It is well known that Siberian ginseng can increase endurance, lessen fatigue, and increase stamina. Athletes and others looking to improve their physical performance commonly use it. Siberian ginseng is also taken by some individuals to increase mental alertness.

Other variations of Ginseng: There are a few less common but potentially beneficial ginseng variations in addition to the more well-known varieties.

Indian ginseng (Ashwagandha), Brazilian ginseng (Suma root), and Peruvian ginseng (Maca root) are a few examples. Improved energy, libido, and general vitality are just a few of the health benefits these kinds are said to give.

They have been employed in the traditional medical systems of their various countries.

It's important to remember that these ginseng variants may have different active ingredients and possible health effects. Thus, while thinking about taking ginseng supplements, it's important to do your homework, select the kind that corresponds with your unique health objectives, and speak with a medical expert to find the best alternative for you.

In addition, it's critical to take ginseng supplements according to the directions and to be informed of any possible negative effects and combinations with other drugs or medical problems.

# CHAPTER THREE

## How To Take Ginseng Supplementally

Due to its possible health benefits, ginseng, a well-known herbal medication, has been utilized in traditional medicine for millennia. It is regarded as an adaptogen, a naturally occurring compound that could support the body's ability to balance and adjust to stress.

Supplements containing ginseng are available in many forms; the two most popular varieties are American ginseng (Panax quinquefolius) and Asian or Korean ginseng (Panax ginseng). The choice to take ginseng as a supplement should be based on the needs and particular health objectives of the user.

Supplements containing ginseng are frequently used to increase vitality, boost energy levels, and improve mental clarity. The active ingredients in ginseng, called ginsenosides, may have some role in these benefits, according to research. These substances may strengthen the immune system and enhance cognitive performance because of their antioxidant and anti-inflammatory qualities. However, individual differences in ginseng supplement efficacy exist, and outcomes cannot be assured.

## The Administration And Dosage

It might be difficult to determine the right amount of ginseng to take as a supplement because it varies on several variables, such as the person's age, sex, weight, and general health.

In general, ginseng supplements come in a variety of formats, with varying amounts of active components, including extracts, pills, and capsules. It is best to begin with a modest dose and raise it gradually while keeping a close eye on how your body reacts.

The suggested dosage varies greatly; some sources propose taking 200–400 mg of standardized ginseng extract or 1-2 grams of dried ginseng root daily. It's crucial to adhere to the manufacturer's recommendations or seek the advice of a medical expert for specific recommendations. Since ginseng may have modest stimulant effects, it is usually taken in the morning to prevent any sleep problems.

## Ginseng In Combination With Other Supplements

It's important to be aware of possible interactions with other supplements or drugs when thinking about taking ginseng supplements. Blood thinners, anti-diabetic medications, and antidepressants are just a few of the medications that ginseng may interact with. Ginseng overstimulation can result from combining it with coffee or other stimulants, which might have negative effects like anxiety, sleeplessness, or elevated heart rate.

To ensure safe and efficient use, it is advised to speak with a healthcare professional before taking ginseng with other supplements or drugs.

A medical expert can offer advice on possible interactions and assist in developing a thorough supplement regimen customized to a person's specific health requirements.

# CHAPTER FOUR

## Possible Adverse Reactions And Safety Measures

Although ginseng is generally thought to be safe when taken as prescribed, certain people may have negative consequences. Insomnia, upset stomachs, and headaches are common adverse effects. Due to the lack of research on ginseng supplements' safety during pregnancy and lactation, care should be taken when using them.

Ginseng may affect blood pressure, thus people with certain medical disorders, including hypertension, should be cautious when consuming it.

Additionally, because ginseng may interfere with blood coagulation, it should be avoided right before surgery.

It's critical to be aware of any ginseng allergies or sensitivities and to stop using the herb if any negative side effects appear. All things considered, ginseng supplementation needs to be handled carefully, and speaking with a healthcare professional is recommended—especially for people who already have medical issues or are worried about possible negative consequences.

## Traditional Medical Uses Of Ginseng

For thousands of years, ginseng has been used in traditional Asian medicine, where it is considered a valuable treatment for a wide range of illnesses.

Ginseng is used as an adaptogen to support general health and is said to replenish vital energy, or "qi," in traditional Chinese medicine. It is regarded as a tonic plant that helps fight weariness, increase mental clarity, and increase stamina.

Similarly, American ginseng is employed for its supposed adaptogenic and immune-boosting qualities in traditional medicine in North America. It has been utilized as a medicine by indigenous tribes to treat a variety of ailments, such as fevers, colds, and stomach problems.

It's important to keep in mind that current scientific study on ginseng is still underway, even if its traditional use in these antiquated medical systems offers insightful information about its possible advantages. Some of the traditional claims have started to be supported by scientific research, however, ginseng's suitability for treating particular medical conditions may differ. Consequently, when using ginseng as a supplement, people should see a healthcare provider. Ginseng should be seen as an adjunct to traditional medical therapies.

## Ginseng in Contemporary Studies

After being used for millennia in traditional medicine, ginseng has attracted a lot of interest in contemporary study. Numerous investigations have been conducted to uncover its secrets since scientists and herbalists have been enthralled with its possible health advantages.

The word "ginseng" usually refers to the roots of plants in the Panax genus, of which Panax ginseng (Asian) and Panax quinquefolius (American) are the two most widely used types.

## Research Studies Concerning Ginseng

Many scientific disciplines, including pharmacology, biochemistry, clinical medicine, and nutrition, have contributed to the investigation of ginseng's potential health benefits. The chemical makeup, pharmacological characteristics, and possible medicinal uses of ginseng are all explored in these studies.

Ginsenosides, polysaccharides, and polyacetylenes are just a few of the bioactive substances found in ginseng's chemical makeup.

Particularly ginsenosides are frequently regarded as the main active ingredients in charge of the herb's biological actions. Scholars have carried out comprehensive examinations to recognize and measure these substances, illuminating the particular elements that contribute to ginseng's health-enhancing attributes.

Studies on pharmacology have explored the possible modes of action of ginseng. These studies have looked into the interactions that ginseng has with many biological systems and pathways, such as the immunological, cardiovascular, and neurological systems. Research on ginseng's adaptogenic qualities—which are thought to aid the body in adjusting to stress and preserving equilibrium—has been primarily focused in this regard.

To fully comprehend the medicinal potential of ginseng, clinical investigations have also been essential.

Scholars have investigated its impact on a range of medical disorders, including but not limited to diabetes, tiredness, and cognitive performance.

Randomized controlled trials are frequently used in these studies to assess the safety and effectiveness of ginseng-based therapies in practical settings.

# CHAPTER FIVE

## The Potential Of Ginseng For Chronic Illnesses

The possibility of ginseng to treat chronic illnesses is one of the most fascinating areas of ginseng research.

Numerous research studies have indicated that ginseng may provide benefits for a range of health conditions, such as diabetes, heart disease, and neurological disorders. For example, it has been discovered that ginsenosides, the bioactive components of ginseng, have anti-diabetic effects via enhancing insulin sensitivity and glucose metabolism.

Moreover, research has been conducted on the potential benefits of ginseng for cardiovascular health.

According to research, ginseng may help lower blood pressure, improve lipid profiles, and strengthen blood vessels. These outcomes may help prevent and treat heart-related conditions like high blood pressure and atherosclerosis.

Research has investigated ginseng's potential to mitigate cognitive decline and memory problems in the context of neurodegenerative illnesses. Because of the herb's neuroprotective qualities, which are believed to be connected to its anti-inflammatory and antioxidant qualities, ginseng may be used in addition to other treatments for diseases including Alzheimer's and age-related cognitive decline.

### Research On Ginseng And Cancer

Because of its potential as an adjuvant therapy, ginseng has also sparked attention in cancer research. Numerous studies have examined ginseng's potential to reduce some of the negative effects of cancer treatment and potentially strengthen the body's natural defenses against the disease, even though it is not a stand-alone cancer treatment.

The immunomodulatory qualities of ginseng have drawn special attention to cancer. Ginsenosides are thought to activate the immune system, which could aid the body in identifying and eliminating cancer cells more successfully.

Additionally, studies have looked into ginseng's potential to lessen cancer-related fatigue, raise patients' quality of life, and increase their general well-being while receiving cancer therapy.

Numerous potential health benefits of ginseng have been revealed during its path from a traditional herbal treatment to a contemporary study focus.

Research on its chemical makeup, pharmacological characteristics, and therapeutic uses has been conducted by scientists; these studies have shown that it has the potential to treat chronic illnesses and aid in the fight against cancer.

Although additional investigation is necessary to completely clarify the scope of its medicinal benefits, ginseng continues to be a fascinating topic in the field of contemporary medicine and health science.

Ginseng in Daily Life: Known for its adaptogenic qualities, ginseng is a powerful herb that has permeated many facets of daily existence. For millennia, it has been an essential component of traditional medicine in many Asian countries.

Because of this amazing plant's possible health benefits, many have started to include it as a nutritional supplement in their everyday routines.

Ginseng is a well-liked option for people looking to increase their energy and fight weariness because it is said to improve general vitality and well-being.

Apart from its usage as a nutritional supplement, ginseng has gained recognition in traditional medicine for its ability to treat a variety of health conditions, including stress management and cognitive function enhancement.

Because of its adaptogenic qualities, ginseng can support the body's ability to adjust to a variety of stimuli and preserve equilibrium. This has made it a beneficial addition to the daily routines of several people who want to boost their mental and physical well-being.

### Ginseng In Culinary Arts:

The use of ginseng in culinary arts demonstrates its adaptability beyond traditional medical uses. Ginseng is regarded as a valued component and delicacy in certain cuisines. With its distinct flavor and slightly bitter taste, ginseng root is frequently used in stews, soups, and other savory meals. Its unique flavor gives a variety of culinary creations depth and complexity.

For example, ginseng is an essential ingredient in traditional Korean cuisines like kimchi, a fermented vegetable dish, and samgyetang, a chicken soup flavored with ginseng flavor. These recipes are not just tasty but also nutrient-dense since ginseng adds not only flavor but also potential health benefits.

# CHAPTER SIX

## Ginseng In Beauty And Skincare:

Ginseng is becoming more and more popular outside of the kitchen and medical cabinet. It is being used in beauty and skincare products. The antioxidant qualities of ginseng root are well-known, and they may aid in preventing free radicals from harming skin cells. As a result, ginseng extracts are now included in a variety of skincare products, such as toners, masks, and serums.

Ginseng is thought to support skin health by lowering inflammation and enhancing circulation.

It is frequently used in skin-brightening and skin-rejuvenating treatments as well as anti-aging creams to lessen the appearance of fine lines and wrinkles. Furthermore, ginseng is an important component in the quest for youthful, glowing skin because of its capacity to increase the creation of collagen.



### Ginseng In Tea And Beverages:

It has long been known that ginseng is a crucial component of many different teas and drinks. Particularly ginseng tea has become very popular due to its distinct flavor and possible health advantages. A common method for making ginseng tea is to steep ginseng root or extracts in hot water to produce a fragrant and energizing beverage.

This drink is well-known for its ability to increase vitality, improve mental clarity, and raise energy levels.

Because ginsenosides, the main ingredients in ginseng, have an energetic impact, it's frequently used as a natural substitute for coffee. Apart from tea, ginseng is often used in herbal infusions, energy drinks, and even alcoholic drinks. It imparts a unique herbal flavor and is occasionally marketed as having stimulating qualities.

Ginseng has a wide-ranging impact on daily life that goes well beyond conventional treatment. Whether used as a dietary supplement, a flavoring agent for drinks, a culinary element, or a skincare ingredient, ginseng never fails to enthrall people with its multifarious applications and possible health and well-being advantages.

## How To Grow And Gather Ginseng

Growing Ginseng: Ginseng, or Panax ginseng, is a highly valued herb that has been used for a very long time in East Asian traditional medicine. This medicinal plant requires particular environmental conditions and requires careful cultivation. Generally speaking, ginseng grows best in temperate woodlands with somewhat shaded, loamy soil that drains well. Selecting the ideal site for production is crucial.

To start, the soil must be prepared by clearing away any rocks, weeds, and other materials that could obstruct the ginseng roots' ability to grow. Growers usually plant ginseng seeds in the early fall after the soil has been sufficiently prepared. This allows the seeds to naturally stratify, which is essential for germination. The next spring, the seeds begin to sprout.

**Gathering And Preserving Ginseng:**
Gathering ginseng requires careful attention to detail and patience. The most prized ginseng roots are at least 5 to 7 years old, and they usually require several years to grow. Typically, the harvesting season occurs

in the early or late summer. Harvesters ensure that the plant is not severely damaged by delicately excavating the roots. Leaving some roots in the earth to yield seeds for future crops is crucial for sustainability.

After being harvested, ginseng roots are dried, cleaned, and graded according to size. Because it keeps the active substances in the root intact and stops mildew and rot, proper drying is essential. To preserve their therapeutic qualities, the dried roots are then kept in a cold, dark, and well-ventilated area.

## Ginseng Conservation Efforts:

Because of the declining natural populations and rising demand for this priceless herb, ginseng conservation is a critical priority. The natural habitats of ginseng are being protected and maintained, and sustainable cultivation is being supported by several programs and organizations.

To stop overharvesting and poaching of this valuable resource, restrictions are being established for the gathering of wild ginseng. When it comes to the U.S. By the Convention on International Trade in Endangered Species of Wild Fauna and Flora (CITES), the Fish and Wildlife Service oversees the trade in wild ginseng. To protect wild ginseng populations, harvesters must get permits and follow stringent requirements.

To increase public knowledge of the value of ginseng conservation, botanic gardens, and conservationists jointly organize educational programs. They support responsible harvesting and sustainable production methods among ginseng growers. To prevent any harm to wild populations, this involves promoting the ethical procurement of ginseng products.

In addition, studies on ginseng cultivation and propagation techniques are being conducted to lessen the strain on wild populations. Reliance on wild ginseng may be lessened through ginseng production in agroforestry systems, where ginseng is planted alongside other forest species.

To produce high-quality roots, growing and harvesting ginseng is a complex procedure that requires time, care, and attention to environmental factors. To ensure that this priceless plant is available for future generations and can be sustainably used in traditional medicine and herbal supplements, conservation activities are essential in preventing overharvesting and habitat loss.

# CHAPTER SEVEN

## The Prospects For Ginseng

Ginseng's future is bright and full of possibilities as this beloved herb continues to draw interest from scientists, health-conscious people, and consumers all around the world.

Traditionally used in Asian cultures, ginseng has a long history in traditional medicine due to its adaptogenic qualities and supposed health advantages. Its increased global renown in recent years can be attributed to the growing interest in complementary and alternative medicine as well as natural therapies.

The trajectory of ginseng's future is intimately linked to the changing field of herbal medicine and scientific inquiry. We should expect a clearer comprehension of the ways via which ginseng affects the human body as new research reveals its medicinal benefits. This could result in the creation of more focused and potent ginseng-based treatments for a range of illnesses, such as stress, weariness, and cognitive decline.

## Ecological Methods

The use of sustainable farming methods is one of the key factors influencing the future of ginseng.

Due to its high demand and sluggish growth rate, ginseng—especially American ginseng (Panax quinquefolius) and Korean ginseng (Panax ginseng—is susceptible to overharvesting.

Reduced numbers of wild ginseng are a concern as a result of unsustainable harvesting practices.

An expanding number of sustainable cultivation and harvesting techniques are being investigated to solve these environmental issues, including organic farming, ginseng cultivated in the shade, and ginseng farmed like that of the wild. Environmentally responsible methods that prioritize securing the herb's long-term availability for future generations will determine the fate of ginseng.

**Prospective Findings And Innovations**
The identification of new chemicals and uses for ginseng is another area with enormous promise for the future. The bioactive elements of ginseng, known as ginsenosides, have been thoroughly investigated; however, more research may uncover new ginsenosides with particular health advantages. Additionally, ginseng's potential

as a component in a variety of formulations—from nutritional supplements to cosmetics—keeps growing.

New developments in biotechnology and pharmacology have made it possible to formulate and extract substances with greater accuracy. This opens the door for improvements in ginseng-based products, increasing their potency and accessibility. For example, ginseng nanotechnology may result in increased bioavailability, hence augmenting its potential therapeutic uses.

## Worldwide Supply And Demand

Ginseng is becoming more and more in demand worldwide due to growing trends in health-conscious consumer behavior, herbal supplements, and traditional medicines. The dynamic relationship between supply and demand will have a big impact on ginseng's future.

North America is a major supplier and consumer of ginseng, with China and South Korea ranking among the top producers and consumers. With more nations looking to take advantage of ginseng's economic potential, the global ginseng market is becoming more and more competitive.

To manage the supply and demand of ginseng while maintaining its ecological and cultural significance, sustainable growing methods, international trade laws, and quality control procedures will be crucial. To preserve the long-term sustainability of the herb and guarantee a steady market, ginseng will need to adopt a balanced strategy in the future.

# Conclusion

Global demand and supply dynamics, possible discoveries and improvements, and sustainable practices will all dynamically interact to shape the future of ginseng. Given its lengthy history and continued scientific study, ginseng is regarded as a major actor in the field of herbal medicine and alternative health care. To guarantee that this amazing plant thrives and continues to improve human well-being for future generations, it is imperative that we carefully control the demand for ginseng, emphasize sustainable growing practices, and make investments in research and innovation.